Turmeric Superfood

Amazing Health Remedies, Cookbook Recipes, and Beauty Treatments

© Copyright 2017 by Vouch Publishing - All rights reserved.

The following eBook is reproduced below with the goal of providing information that is as accurate and reliable as possible. Regardless, purchasing this eBook can be seen as consent to the fact that both the publisher and the author of this book are in no way experts on the topics discussed within and that any recommendations or suggestions that are made herein are for entertainment purposes only. Professionals should be consulted as needed prior to undertaking any of the action endorsed herein.

This declaration is deemed fair and valid by both the American Bar Association and the Committee of Publishers Association and is legally binding throughout the United States.

Furthermore, the transmission, duplication or reproduction of any of the following work including specific information will be considered an illegal act irrespective of if it is done electronically or in print. This extends to creating a secondary or tertiary copy of the work or a recorded copy and is only allowed with express written consent from the Publisher. All additional right reserved. The information in the following pages is broadly considered to be a truthful and accurate account of facts and as such any inattention, use or misuse of the information in question by the reader will render any resulting actions solely under their purview. There are no scenarios in which the publisher or the original author of this work can be in any fashion deemed liable for any hardship or damages that may befall them after undertaking information described herein.

Additionally, the information in the following pages is intended only for informational purposes and should thus be thought of as universal. As befitting its nature, it is presented without assurance regarding its prolonged validity or interim quality. Trademarks that are mentioned are done without written consent and can in no way be considered an endorsement from the trademark holder.

Some elements of the front book cover were designed by Planolla / Freepik.

Thanks for purchasing this book!

*As a thank you, we'd love to offer you another amazing eBook for FREE
Visit the link below to grab your unrestricted free copy…*

http://bit.ly/myvouchgift

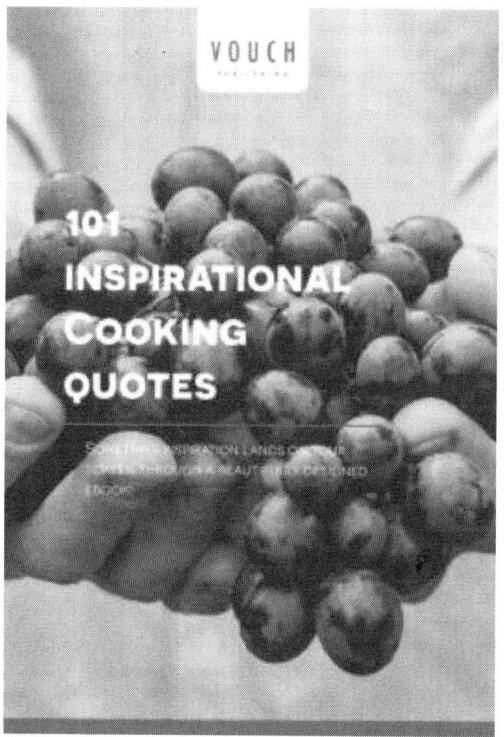

101 Inspirational Cooking Quotes

Inside this free eBook, you will find amazing quotes from famous awe-inspiring people who love to cook just like me and you!

Table of Contents

Introduction 6
Chapter 1: What is Turmeric? 8
    Where does Turmeric Originate from? 8
    Chemical Composition of Turmeric 8
    Ways to Use Turmeric 9
    Curcumin Elements 10
    Turmeric Root vs Powder Form 10
    Possible Side Effects 11
Chapter 2: How Turmeric Works 13
    Ailments that Benefit from Turmeric 13
    Health Benefits in Comparison 17
    The Research Says It All 18
Chapter 3: Turmeric 'Golden Paste' Medicinal Remedies 21
    How to Prepare the 'Golden Paste' 21
    Daily Supplement Booster 22
    Additional Ways to Use the 'Golden Paste' 24
    Benefits for Horses & Pets 26
Chapter 4: Turmeric Cookbook Recipes 29
    Breakfast Recipes 30
    Chicken Recipes 34
    Beef Recipes 40
    Side Dishes, Soups & Salads 44
    Snacks & Sauces 56
Chapter 5: Turmeric Rich Warm Beverages 64
    Warm Drinks 65
    Turmeric Tea Golden Milk Recipe 65
    Turmeric Tea Mix 66
    Apple and Green Turmeric Tea (Cold and Flu Tonic) 67
    Turmeric Coffee 69
    Honey and Turmeric Latte 70
    Turmeric Hot Chocolate 71

Spiced Matcha Latte 72
Chapter 6: Shakes and Smoothies 73
Chapter 7: Quick-Fix Turmeric Beauty Mixtures 77
    Healthy Hair and Skin 77
    Use as a Mask or Wash 78
    Words of Caution... 81
Chapter 8: Beautiful Homemade Skin Treatments 83
    Neck Area Concoction #1: Gram Flour, Cream and Turmeric Pack.. 84
    Face Cleanse Concoction #2: Turmeric, Almond and Milk Pack 85
    Blackheads Concoction #3: Turmeric and Egg White......................... 86
    Acne Concoction #4: The Acne Prone Skin Pack 87
    Deep Cleaner Concoction#5: Lemon Juice, Turmeric and Gram Flour 88
    Oily & Dry Skin Concoction #6: Turmeric, Honey and Cornstarch Pack 89
    Ultimate Face Lift Concoction #7: The Ultimate Turmeric Face Pack.. 90
    Directions 90
    Cooling Off Concoction #8: Chill Out with Fuller's Earth 91
    Itchy Skin Concoction #9: Turmeric and Oatmeal Aids Irritation 91
    Dandruff Concoction #10: Dandruff Treatment 92
    Toothpaste Concoction #11: Amazing Turmeric Toothpaste 92
Conclusion 94
Index 97

Introduction

Congratulations on purchasing your personal copy of the Turmeric Benefits and Cookbook Recipes. Thank you for doing so. You will better understand the many benefits of this common ingredient found within the Indian style of cooking. It is best known in the United States as a spice and one of the main components of curry powder.

Many health conditions have also been treated in India as well as other parts of Southeast Asia for several thousands of years dating back to the Ayurvedic tradition (holistic or whole body healing systems).

This 'spice' has amazing antioxidant, anti-inflammatory and, believe it or not, anticancer properties as well. You will discover how great turmeric is as a spice which comes from rhizomes or underground stems of the turmeric plant. The spice also helps retain the beta-carotene in some foods such as pumpkins and carrots.

These are some of the ways we will explore to provide you with necessary information so you can remedy some of your health ailments. Here are of that long list:

- Obesity

- Alzheimer's disease
- Arthritis
- Blood Pressure is Lowered
- Bowel Disease
- Cystic Fibrosis
- Lowered Cholesterol Levels are Lowered
- Depression
- Diabetes
- Heart Protection
- Immunity Booster
- A Healthier Liver
- Uveitis

There are plenty of books on this subject on the market, thanks again for choosing this one! Every effort was made to ensure it is full of as much useful information as possible for you to understand fully all aspects of this exotic spice.

Please enjoy!

Chapter 1: What is Turmeric?

Where does Turmeric Originate from?

The species of genus Curcuma called Curcuma longa Linn is better known as the species of turmeric. These are some of its shared and Indian names: Arasina (Kananda), Halad (Marathi), Haldi (Hindi), Haldar (Gujarati), Pasupu (Telugu), Manjal (Tamil), Halud (Bengali), and Manjal (Malayalam).

The herb has no stems but has tuberous root stalks which are stalk-like and long. To grow it needs an abundance of rainfall with temperatures ranging between 20° and 30° to flourish.

Chemical Composition of Turmeric

The leaves are generally close to two feet tall, but the tubers and rhizomes are used in the turmeric powder. The following is the chemical composition of turmeric:

- Carbohydrates = 69.4%
- Protein = 6.3%
- Mineral matter = 3.5%
- Moisture = 3.1%
- Fiber = 2.6%

- Fat = 5.1%

Ways to Use Turmeric

There are quite a few ways in which you can use turmeric. It's actually really simple to start introducing this classic medicinal spice into your diet so you can start reaping the benefits of it! Here are just a few:

- You could prepare some brown rice with cashews and raisins; season with some coriander, cumin, and turmeric.

- Give your egg salad a fancy yellowish shade.
- When preparing curries, you can add a little extra for an additional kick.

- Add it to your salads and smoothies, which are already a healthy choice but are made better with turmeric.
Several recipes and ideas are mentioned throughout the book to give you new ways to make your life healthier. These prior examples are just a tasting of what is to come later! Believe me, throughout the course of this book, you are going to be absolutely flooded with completely and totally delicious turmeric recipes that will make your mouth water and make you feel, in time, like a million bucks.

Curcumin Elements

Known for its inflammation reduction factors, curcumin is a substance found in turmeric. Studies have uncovered that it can ease symptoms of rheumatoid arthritis and osteoarthritis.

As a result of lab testing, the curcumin aspect of turmeric appears to block some types of tumors. One particular study indicated colorectal cancer that was not helped by prior treatments using other methods was improved with the treatments from the extract—curcumin.

Turmeric Root vs Powder Form

In its natural form, turmeric is an orange, knobby root which looks very similar to ginger. You can purchase turmeric fresh as a root from various places including on Amazon's website.

If you want to purchase it in its root form and manually transform it into powder yourself then you will need to go through the following time consuming process:

- Sweating
- Curing
- Drying
- Grinding

Don't forget, you can use both the root and the powder form for your cooking needs. Although, sometimes it can be much simpler to use the powdered form which can be purchased at most convenient stores. The rule-of-thumb is a ratio of 1 to 3. Therefore, one teaspoon of dried spice equals three teaspoons or one tablespoon of the freshly grated spice. For a two-inch chunk of fresh root; you will yield one tablespoon of fresh grated turmeric.

Possible Side Effects

Turmeric is naturally grown and considered a safe product. It is said that for some people in higher doses or long-term usage; it could cause some nausea or diarrhea and some minor skin irritation. From my research, there have been no reports of any significant or severe side effects involved with the use of turmeric, whether applied or ingested.

According to Ben Franklin, "An ounce of prevention is worth a pound of cure." Many times, symptoms are noticed if you use too much before your body has a chance to adjust. It is just one minor element that should be considered.

The symptoms should pass as you become accustomed to the changes in your diet. If it is a reaction to a concoction placed on your skin; simply — stop using the product. It can also be a reaction to other medications you may be taking. If the symptoms don't reside, you should check with your physician. Lastly, if you intend to use it alongside your current medication, you should speak to your doctor or physician as a precaution.

Chapter 2: How Turmeric Works

There are a lot of benefits that come from incorporating this miraculous spice into your diet. Turmeric is an excellent source of manganese as well as vitamin B6, potassium, fiber, and copper.

If you have a chronic condition – mental or physical – there's a good chance that turmeric will help you in one way or another. Read on to find out the various ailments which turmeric can help with – you'll find that there are probably more than you expected!

Ailments that Benefit from Turmeric

Obesity: Research has indicated that the curcumin element within turmeric can break down fat cells and stop them in their path quickly. Couple that with a healthier diet; you have a 'win-win' situation.

Arthritis: If you suffer from muscle and joint pain and take over-the-counter medications; turmeric may be the answer to your problem. The free radicals are reduced by the release of curcumin which helps your muscles and bones work as they should. The spice has the same effects of the likes of phenylbutazone and hydrocortisone. But remember that it is advisable to consult your physician before you experiment with your medications.

Alzheimer's: Turmeric has shown promising signs in the prevention of this dreaded disease that can cripple a person as well as their entire family. It is plagued by the brain not being able to process insulin as energy. Its side effects can include extreme forgetfulness along with changing the person's general character.

Blood Pressure: You can stop the oxidation of the harmful cholesterol that forms in the body. It protects from plaque buildup which causes the pressure to rise. The oxidized cholesterol can cause blood clots that will make it impossible to lower the pressure. Preventative maintenance using turmeric, along with some engaging cardio, is essential.

Bowel Disease: Crohn's, irritable bowel syndrome, colitis, and ulcerative colitis sufferers could also benefit from symptom reduction by consuming more turmeric. This spice will help your digestive system function better and allow your cells to work as they should without interruption.

Cystic Fibrosis: Lab research has discovered curcumin

can help to correct lung defects. They also suggest that the substance could reduce the difficulties in breathing as well as reduce some of the side effects that come along with this disorder. Individuals who are currently using turmeric as part of their treatment plan have provided encouraging results.

Cancer Prevention: The symptoms of some cancers can be eased with the use of turmeric spice. A study in 2006, for individuals who were born with precancerous polyps in the colon, indicated that if you consume turmeric on a regular basis you could decrease the size of them by more than sixty percent. The nature of this spice helps prevent cellular damage which can potentially cause cancer to form.

Cholesterol: Along with a diet of reduced saturated fats, adding turmeric can help lower high cholesterol levels in the body. Curcumin helps stop cell growth in the liver and prevent the creation of 'bad' cholesterol and then redirects the growth to create the 'good' cholesterol. The combination of turmeric with a healthy lifestyle can help speed up the process.

Depression: Depression can be caused by depleted or imbalanced neurotransmitters inside the body. This part's a bit technical but turmeric aids the monoamine oxidase (MAO) enzymes which prevent the neurotransmitter depletion and boosts the dopamine and serotonin to restore the levels. This process is called neurogenesis.

Diabetes: The use of turmeric helps moderate your insulin levels. It may also prevent the onset of type-2 diabetes by reducing your insulin resistance.

Note: Consult a healthcare professional if you currently take strong medications before consuming turmeric as a form of medication because it could cause low blood sugar (hypoglycemia), even though these cases are rare.

Heart Disease: Vitamin B is supplied by turmeric which is essential to your body to prevent homocysteine levels from becoming too excessive. Research has proven that individuals who consume more curcumin (i.e. turmeric) will most likely experience improved blood vessel and heart health.

Immunity Booster: Lipopolysaccharide is a substance found in turmeric that helps to stimulate your immune system. You will have less chance of suffering from coughs, flu, and colds. One quick remedy for you is to drink a glass of hot milk once daily with one teaspoon of turmeric powder.

Liver: Curcumin can also prevent liver cirrhosis. The

natural chemicals that turmeric provides, according to research in Israel, can help heal damaged liver tissues.

Uveitis: The middle layer of tissue on the eye wall (uvea) can have an eye inflammation called uveitis. Since turmeric is beneficial for inflammation, it can also help with some of the symptoms of this vision ailment that can lead to blindness. Once again, discuss this with your doctor or your optometrist if you are concerned.

Health Benefits in Comparison

According to 6,235 peer-viewed articles in the US National Library of Medicine and the National Institutes of Health, the following drugs pale compared to turmeric:

- Painkillers
- Anti-inflammatory drugs
- Cholesterol drugs (Lipitor)
- Antidepressants (Prozac)
- Diabetes medications
- Chemotherapy
- Arthritis medications
- Steroids
- Inflammatory Bowel disease drugs

The Research Says It All

As stated previously, studies have been given to provide you with related incidents where varieties of individuals have benefited from turmeric and, it's essential compound, curcumin. These are a few of those stories:

Anti-depressants: The journal *Phytotherapy Research* published study results where sixty volunteers that were diagnosed with major depressive disorder (or MDD). The group was split into patients who were taking Prozac, turmeric/curcumin, and a mishmash of the two. It was revealed that the curcumin was just as effective in managing depression as the Prozac. It was a huge breakthrough towards providing 'clinical' evidence for the spice and its benefits.

Arthritis Management: A study was conducted using 45 patients who had rheumatoid arthritis who were currently taking medications such as diclofenac sodium. The drug is known for placing patients at risk of heart disease or developing a leaky gut. Once again, three groups were provided with different elements; one had the curcumin treatment, one used the diclofenac sodium alone, and the last group was given a combination of the two.

Guess the results? If you guessed the highest percentage shown from the Disease Activity Score was from the curcumin group; you are correct! The patients suffered no adverse effects.

Anti-inflammatory: *Oncogene Journal* published some astonishing results from studies comparing ibuprofen and aspirin with the benefits of curcumin. As a consequence of these studies, diseases such as the above mentioned as well as chronic pain sufferers who may also have symptoms from uncreative colitis and cancer; also, discovered the benefits resulting in less inflammation. In each of these cases; turmeric is the key to disease reversal with its many abilities to keep your inflammation and pain at bay.

Oily Skin Corrected: You could be suffering from overactive sebaceous glands which can lead to skin conditions such as acne or cysts. A study in 2012, which was documented by the Tropical Journal of Pharmaceutical Research, discovered a decrease in skin oils over a four-week treatment plan when turmeric was applied twice daily. After three months, facial oils had almost reached 25% improvements which were most likely because of the phytosterols and fatty acids in the turmeric.

Prevention of Skin Cancer: Studies were provided in 1998, and another in 2011, providing a wealth of information that curcumin was able to produce cell death and, in some cases, prevented the cells from forming.

Chapter 3: Turmeric 'Golden Paste' Medicinal Remedies

How to Prepare the 'Golden Paste'

You can acquire the benefits of turmeric in many ways. These are just a few of the ways you can achieve these goals by using a plan because the paste can indeed deliver incredible benefits. This is how to make your batch of homemade paste, so that you can begin your own adventure with turmeric:

Ingredients for the 'Golden Paste'
1 cup of water
2-3 tsp. black pepper (freshly ground)
½ cup turmeric powder
1/3 cup of one of the following of your choice:
- Linseed/flaxseed oil
- Extra virgin olive oil
- Raw unrefined coconut oil

Directions
1) Bring the water and turmeric close to boiling; lower the heat and continue cooking slowly until a thick paste is formed. The process should take 7 to 10

minutes. You can add small amounts of water if necessary.
2) Add the pepper and oil after the cooking phase is completed (after it has cooled to just warm).
3) Stir well and allow it to cool. Refrigerate and consume the 'Golden Paste' within 2 weeks. You can also freeze a portion of the paste, if you do not believe you can use it within that time.

Daily Supplement Booster

This homemade dosage is easier to swallow, so it is better for children.

Ingredients
1/3 cup organic ground turmeric
1 Tbsp. quercetin powder (10 – emptied capsules)
Big pinch of black pepper (finely ground)
Binding Agent: Chose from the following — 3 Tbsp. total needed
- Coconut oil
- Raw honey
- Grass-fed ghee

Directions
1) Use some unbleached parchment paper to line a baking sheet. Clean out space in the freezer for the

bombs to rest and set for several hours.
2) Wear an apron and protect your counters since turmeric powder has a tendency to stain clothing.
3) *The Binding Agents:* You need three agents total. If you choose ghee, coconut oil, or the raw honey; you may need to melt them over low heat until it's pourable (not hot).
4) Combine the pepper, turmeric, binding agent, and quercetin in a mixing bowl.
5) Honey will be pliable and thick; so, pinch the dough between your palms and roll it. For the oil binder; you should have a more viscous mixture to form easily into a pill.

The above ingredients increase the bioavailability of the previously mentioned curcumin — the anti-inflammatory compound found in turmeric.

Here's how they work:

1) Fatty acids have been shown to increase the bioavailability of the source of turmeric.
2) Black pepper also contains potent alkaloid piperine which also enhances the bioavailability up to 150 percent.
3) Quercetin which is a bioflavonoid also inhibits an enzyme that will decrease the activity of the

curcumin.

Use the bombs as needed: If you are using the honey version, remember, it has some sugar. On the other hand, don't take a lot of the oil-based version because it could upset your stomach. You can adjust the dosage as you go.

Yields: Around 50 bombs

Additional Ways to Use the 'Golden Paste'

Take it Solo: Take the paste in small quantities up to 2 to 3 times each day.

Add some Honey: Manuka honey is considered by many to be the best type. When adding honey, make sure it is pure. Just mix the paste and honey; down the hatch!

Use some Fruits: You can use the paste with dried fruits by warming it on the stovetop and adding it to your choice of fruit.

Add to Warm Milk: Warm milk will induce the sleep.
1) Adding a ½-to one-inch piece of turmeric with eight ounces of milk is the first step. Heat it up to 15 minutes. Strain the turmeric and drink it after it

cooks to soothe diarrhea, inflammation, and strengthen the bones.

2) *Use it as a mask or wash*: Add ½ teaspoon of ground turmeric to ¼ cup of whole milk. Use a clean cloth and soak it in the mixture. Apply it to the affected skin and leave it on for 10 minutes before you wash it off.

3) *Soothe Coughs and Sore Throats*: Just one sip of turmeric milk can improve your symptoms by morning.
    a. Add 1 teaspoon of minced ginger to ¼ cup of water, and ½ teaspoon of turmeric.
    b. Top off the cup with some milk.
    c. Boil or heat in the microwave until you see the milk is ready to boil.
    d. Let the blends steep for a few minutes. You can add sugar, honey, or cane sugar to your liking. Combine and reheat the mixture for several minutes.
    e. Strain the pieces of turmeric and ginger out of the drink and sip while it is piping hot. If you like pepper, throw the peppercorns in to fully improve the absorption rates of the turmeric into your body.
    f. Add a pinch of saffron and a few pods of cracked cardamom to the water/milk concoction before you boil the ingredients.

Benefits for Horses & Pets

The paste is good for humans, but don't leave out the other critters such as horses, dogs, and cats. These are some of the other ways you can use the Golden Paste:

If necessary/needed, you can increase the amount used after every 5 days. Your animals will require a slightly different formula:

Horses

Ingredients
1 tsp. Golden Paste
2 tsp. turmeric powder
16 grinds ground black peppercorns
2 tsp. oil

Directions
The maximum dosage is 1 to 2 tablespoons of the paste at one time, and normally 2 teaspoons will do the trick.

Horses will usually accept the turmeric powder to the feed, but you need to add the amounts gradually. If you choose to feed it to your horse through the feed, the ratio is 1 teaspoon per cup twice daily and you can build it up to a tablespoon spoon full 1 or 2 times each day.
It is given as:
- 1 dessert spoon (10 ml) of the turmeric powder

- 6 to 8 grinds of black peppercorns
- 1 to 2 tsp. linseed, coconut or olive oil

The product can be fed dry or blended into a paste. Experiment with your horse to see if the horse prefers the dry or wet product. You can also offer some baked treats. Horses love a special treat any time!

Pets

Turmeric Treat

Ingredients
1 cup gluten-free self-rising flour
½ cup cooked brown rice
2 eggs
Turmeric powder (recommended dosage in table below)
¼ tsp. ground pepper
½ tsp. coconut oil
½ cup cooked mashed pumpkin

Directions
Preheat the oven to 450°F. Prepare the rice and pumpkin and set to the side.
1) Mix the rice, pumpkin, and eggs along with the oil, pepper, and turmeric according to the doses for your pet.
2) Make the dough by adding flour, a little at a time.

3) Roll the dough out on a board and cut into some original shapes placing them on an oiled baking sheet.
4) Spray a little cooking oil over the tops or drizzle with some coconut oil for the golden finish.
5) Bake for about 10 minutes; give them a flip and cook for another 5 minutes or so.

Note: If humidity is an issue in your area; keep the biscuits in the freezer and thaw as needed.

Weight of the Pet	Turmeric Dosage
5 to 10 Pounds	A pinch to 1/16 tsp.
11 to 20 Pounds	1/16 to 1/8 tsp.
21 to 40 Pounds	1/8 to ¼ tsp.
41 to 80 Pounds	¼ to ½ tsp.
81 to 160 Pounds	½ to 1 tsp.

Chapter 4: Turmeric Cookbook Recipes

One element you need to take into consideration when you begin to cook with turmeric is the importance or organic fresh foods. To receive the best 'boost' for the effort of preparing your healthier meals; you should attempt to use 'wild-caught' or 'free-range' chicken eggs when possible. The additional expense will produce a healthier, more fulfilling product.

Breakfast Recipes

Turmeric and Onion Omelet

Enjoy your eggs with a twist of onion and turmeric to get your day going.

Ingredients
2 finely chopped green onions
4 large eggs
1 Tbsp. olive oil
1/8 tsp. turmeric
¼ tsp. brown mustard seeds
¼ cup diced plum tomato
3/8 tsp. salt
1 dash of ground black pepper

Directions
1) Whisk the eggs and salt together.
2) Prepare a cast-iron skillet with the oil using the stovetop medium-high setting.
3) Add the turmeric and mustard seeds — cooking until the seeds begin popping — stirring frequently.
4) Toss in the onions and continue to stir for about 30 seconds; add the tomato and stir another minute.
5) Empty the egg mixture into the pan and cook for approximately 2 minutes until the edges begin to

cook. Work the egg into the pan's surface using the spatula. Cook until the center is set — usually about 2 minutes or so.
6) Loosen the edges and fold it in half placing it on the platter. Enjoy!

Yields: 2 servings

Suitable for vegetarians

Persian Herb Frittata (Kuku Sabzi)

You can kick back and enjoy this one, and reap the benefits the turmeric has to offer.

Ingredients
½ tsp. turmeric
6 large eggs
1 crushed garlic clove
Pinch of ground black pepper
½ tsp. salt
1 Tbsp. flour
1 cup chopped each:
- Green onions/chives
- Parsley
- Cilantro
- Dill

Optional: 2 Tbsp. each:
- Chopped walnuts
- Vegetable oil/butter/ghee/clarified butter
- Dried cranberries, currants, barberries
- *To Serve: Plain Yogurt*

Directions
Set the oven to 400F. You will need an oven-proof skillet for the eggs.

1) Whisk the cracks of black pepper, eggs, flour, salt and turmeric; add in the walnuts/dried fruit (if using), and herbs.
2) Over moderate heat in a 10 to 12-inch skillet, heat the oil/butter.
3) Empty the mixture into the pan and cook for about 2 minutes or until the edges begin to cook.
4) Place the skillet in the oven to bake for about 5 minutes or until done.
5) Slice the frittata into wedges and garnish hot or cold with a dollop of the yogurt.

Yields: 6 servings

Suitable for vegetarians

Chicken Recipes

Coconut Turmeric Chicken (Slow-Cooker)

This is a delightful recipe blending coconut with the slow cooking method. You will have a hard time waiting for dinner!

Ingredients
1 whole organic chicken
2-inch knob of grated fresh turmeric
½ cup full-fat coconut milk
4 peeled and grated garlic cloves
2-inch knob of grated fresh ginger
Pepper and sea salt
Garnish: Scallions

Directions
1) Be sure to remove the giblets from the chicken and save it for stock.
2) Combine the turmeric, ginger, milk, and garlic in the bottom of the slow cooker.
3) Flavor the chicken with the pepper and salt — inside and out.
4) Sit the bird in the cooker and pour some of the mixture over its surface.
5) Place the lid on the cooker and let it cook on low for 6 to 8 hours or if you prefer, over high for 4 hours.

6) When the bird is done, pull the meat away from the bone and put it into the pot with the juices. Stir it around.
7) Enjoy this over some mashed potatoes, cauliflower puree or rice.

Yields: 2 to 4 servings
Preparation Time: 5 minutes

Ginger Turmeric Chicken

If you enjoy chicken with a kick of ginger, you will love this one.

Ingredients
5-pound Chicken
1 ½ tsp. turmeric or one-inch chunk (fresh)
2-inch piece fresh ginger
2 tsp. salt (or himalayan salt)
2 pressed/grated garlic cloves

Instructions
1) Dry the chicken with some paper towels. Discard the towels and wash your hands.
2) Begin by grating a 1-inch chunk of fresh turmeric and a 2-inch round of ginger. Combine the remainder of the spices and massage over the chicken on the inside and outside.
3) Tie the chicken wings behind the thighs with some kitchen twine.
4) Cook for 15 minutes per pound if you are cooking using the spit on the rotisserie. If cooking in the oven, use the temperature setting of 400°F.
5) Place the chicken on a lined baking dish with the breast facing up until the internal temperature reaches 170°F. at the thickest part of the thigh.

6) Remove it from the oven to rest for about 10 minutes. You can place a towel or piece of parchment paper over the top.

Note: You can save the bones and leftovers for some healthy bone broth later.

Yields: 4 to 6 servings
Preparation Time: 10 minutes
Cooking Time: 75 minutes

Curried Chicken Pasta Salad

A salad for lunch with this one packs heart-healthy and anti-aging benefits.

Ingredients
2 Tbsp. (or ½ ounce) of slivered almonds
2 cups cooked chicken (one-inch pieces)
12 ounces' whole wheat pasta shells
½ cup reduced-fat mayonnaise
1 Tbsp. curry powder
½ cup reduced-fat sour cream or low-fat plain yogurt
1 tsp. turmeric
1/3 cup mango chutney
Pinch of cayenne pepper and salt
¼ tsp. ground cinnamon
½ cup chopped scallions (four)
½ cup diced celery
½ cup raisins

Directions
1) Prepare the pasta in salted water for about 10 minutes—drain—and sit it to the side.
2) Over low heat, toast the almonds in a dry skillet while stirring—approximately 2 minutes or so.
3) Remove and place the pasta in a container to cool.
4) Add the curry to the pan and toast for 30 seconds

using low heat; add it to a small dish. Blend in the yogurt, cinnamon, turmeric, ground red pepper, yogurt, chutney, and mayonnaise.
5) In a large serving bowl; mix the reserved pasta, scallions, chicken, raisins, and celery.
6) If desired — top it off with some almonds.

Notes: For the Poached Chicken Breasts:
1) Use skinless and boneless chicken breasts. Place them in a pan of salted water and bring them to a boil.
2) Cover and lower the heat to cook; boiling them for about 10 to 12 minutes.
3) It is ready for the recipe.
4) Put the bone broth in the freezer for later use.

Yields: 6 servings

Beef Recipes

Spiced Zucchini Beef

This spicy dish is sure to please your crowd and they will never know it is good for your health.

Ingredients
14 ounces minced beef
1 Tbsp. olive oil
½ tsp. ground cumin
½ tsp. turmeric
Pinch of cayenne pepper
1 tsp. ground paprika
2 small to medium zucchini
1 Tbsp. maca powder (also called Peruvian ginseng)
½ tsp. fennel seeds
3 Tbsp. sesame seeds
Pinch of salt
Pinch of pepper

Garnish with a pinch of: Salt, ground cumin, turmeric

Directions
1) Slice the zucchini into rounds.
2) Pour the oil into a skillet and add the beef, cooking on the med-high setting until the beef is cooked.

3) Toss the cumin, cayenne pepper, turmeric, and paprika into the beef and cook for two minutes. Add the zucchini and cook until it wilts, usually about 6 to 8 minutes
4) Take the pan off of the burner for 2 minutes, uncovered, so the beef can slightly cool. Add the pepper, salt, and maca powder.
5) *To Garnish*: Using a small dish, combine the fennel seeds, sesame seeds, cumin, and turmeric. Sprinkle with the mixture and enjoy.

Yields: 2 servings

Original Beef Curry

This spicy dish is sure to please your crowd and they will never know it is good for your health.

Ingredients
2-pounds boneless beef (chopped into 1 inch pieces)
1 cup water
3 Tbsp. olive oil
1 chopped onion
5 cloves of diced garlic
3 green chili peppers
½ a piece of diced ginger
4 cardamom seeds
½ tsp. cinnamon powder
1 tsp. turmeric powder
1 tsp. ground cumin
1 tsp. ground coriander
½ tsp. garlic powder

Directions
1) Put the olive oil in a skillet and set it on medium heat.
2) Add the chopped onion and stir until soft for around 5 minutes. Reduce heat a little and continue cooking for around 15 minutes until dark brown.
3) Add in the diced garlic, sliced green chilies, diced ginger, cardamom seeds and cinnamon powder.

Cook until garlic begins to look brown for around 4 to 6 minutes more.

4) Add the ground cumin, ground coriander, turmeric powder, garlic powder and water into the skillet. Cook until most of the water has gone and the ingredients have become thicker.
5) Add the beef; and let it cook over medium-low heat.
6) Stir the mixture occasionally, until you can see that the beef is thoroughly cooked and tender for about 60 to 90 minutes, depending on your liking.

Yields: 4 to 6 servings
Preparation Time: 30 minutes
Cooking Time: 100 minutes

Side Dishes, Soups & Salads

Freestyle Rice Using Turmeric Paste

This healthy dish is an excellent way to get a good dose of turmeric and fix what is ailing you!

Ingredients
2 cups basmati rice
1 Tbsp. lemon juice
Virgin coconut oil
½ tsp. brown sugar
1 chicken stock cube
Fish sauce (to taste)
2 beaten eggs
2 garlic cloves (crushed or chopped)
1 brown/red chopped onion
1 medium sliced carrot
1 green/red chopped bell pepper
¼ cup corn niblets
½ cup chopped broccoli
¼ cup peas

Directions
1) Use a wok to heat the oil and eggs using medium heat until they are barely cooked. Transfer the eggs to a dish and set to the side.

2) Add a bit more oil if needed; combine the garlic, carrot, and onion. Stir fry until softened.
3) Add the rest of the veggies — stir — and add the stock cube, sugar, juice, and fish sauce still using medium heat for approximately 1 minute.
4) Blend the egg and rice in and mix well until the rice is warmed.
5) Add the paste to each bowl and complement it with some fresh ground pepper.

Yields: 2 to 4 servings

Turmeric Barley-Arugula Salad

This is such a tasty salad to enjoy any time of the day to help with all of your aches and pains.

Ingredients

3 Tbsp. turmeric powder

4 ounces' barley

¾ ounces pumpkin seeds

2 handfuls arugula

15 sliced olives

15 (halved) cherry tomatoes

Olive oil and salt as desired

Directions

1) Prepare a pot of water (8.5 ounces) and one teaspoon of salt using high heat.
2) After it begins to boil; toss in the barley. Once the liquid is absorbed from the 'top' of the pan, reduce the heat and cover the pot. Continue cooking until the water is gone.
3) Remove it from the burner and add the turmeric powder — stir well.
4) In a separate container, combine the tomatoes, seeds, and olives — mixing well.
5) Mix it all together.

6) Add to a bed of arugula and sprinkle with some of the oil.

Yields: 1 to 2 servings

Suitable for vegetarians & vegans

Turmeric Rice

It has never been simpler to take your medicine than it is with this delicious bowl of rice.

Ingredients
2 cups chicken bouillon/water
1 tsp. turmeric
1 cup rice
1 to 2 tsp. butter

Directions
1) Put all of the ingredients into a pan and bring to a boil.
2) Let the rice cook covered and cook slowly for about 15 minutes.
3) Leave it in the pan 5 minutes after the cooking time has elapsed to absorb the flavors.

Yields: 4 to 6 servings

Skillet Gnocchi with White Beans and Turmeric

This recipe is a high-fiber punch for healthy immunity and aging benefits.

Ingredients
1 Tbsp. olive oil
1 thinly sliced medium onion
¼ tsp. turmeric
1- (16 ounce) package gnocchi (shelf-staple)
6 cups (or 1 small bunch) chopped chard leaves/spinach
1 (15 ounce) tinned can rinsed white beans
1 (15 ounce) tinned can diced tomatoes with Italian seasonings
½ cup shredded part-skim mozzarella cheese
¼ tsp. ground pepper
¼ cup parmesan cheese (finely shredded)

Directions
1) Over medium heat, add 1 tablespoon of oil to a skillet. Add the gnocchi—often stirring—for about 2 minutes.
2) Blend in the water and garlic cooking until soft—approximately 4 to 6 minutes.
3) Add the chard to the mixture for a minute or two until it begins to wilt.
4) Pour in the beans, tomatoes, and the important

additional ingredient, the pepper, to activate the turmeric.
5) Blend it all together and stir until the cheeses have melted; around 3 minutes or so.

Note: The gnocchi can be located in the Italian section in most superstores.

Yields: 1 to 2 servings

Suitable for vegetarians

Roasted Turmeric Cauliflower

The turmeric adds special enhancement to this cauliflower dish.

Ingredients
2 tsp. turmeric
2 Tbsp. olive oil
Half head of a large cauliflower
2 tsp. of salt

Directions
1) Set the heat setting in the oven in advance to 350ºF.
2) Remove the florets and add them to a dish with the olive oil, salt, and turmeric.
3) Position the cauliflower in a single layer on a baking sheet/dish and bake for about 75 minutes.

Yields: 1 to 2 servings

Suitable for vegetarians & vegans

Spicy Turmeric Lentils for Salads and Wraps

This mixture is a healthy boost full of high-protein counts, high fiber, as well as anti-oxidant-rich. It will remove the body toxins to help reduce inflammation and maintain a healthy weight.

Ingredients (for the Lentils)
1 cup brown or green lentils
1 sliced garlic clove
½ tsp. salt
1 Tbsp. olive oil
1 tsp. turmeric
1 tsp. marjoram
1 tsp. ground chili powder
1 tsp. cumin

Ingredients (for the Pitas) (normal/medium sized pitas)
Veggies:
- Cucumber
- Tomato
- Spring onions
- Parsley/Basil

Directions
1) Soak the lentils overnight.
2) Prepare the soaked lentils with two cups of water

over medium heat in a large pan with the salt.
3) After the pot boils; lower the heat and cook for ten to twelve minutes. There should be at least 1/3 cups of water left; if not add it.
4) Blend the marjoram, chili powder, turmeric, and garlic to the lentils.
5) Turn the burner off and add the oil.

For the Pitas: Fill them with about 2 tablespoons of the lentil mixture along with some of the desired toppings. Enjoy.

Yields: 1 to 2 servings

Suitable for vegetarians & vegans

Turmeric Butternut Squash Soup

If you have some squash in the garden, this is a tempting treat everyone can enjoy for lunch or dinner.

Ingredients
1 heating tsp. turmeric
2 Tbsp. fresh ginger
1 large butternut squash
1 diced onion
1 can coconut milk (13.66-ounce size)
2 cups vegetable stock (or chicken stock)
1 Tbsp. butter/olive oil/coconut oil
Add salt & pepper to your taste

Optional for Serving:
- Fresh cilantro
- Pumpkin seeds
- Roasted squash seeds

Directions
1) Prepare the squash. Peel and chop the ginger.
2) Using medium heat; sauté the onion and ginger for about 3 minutes.
3) Pour in the stock bringing it to a boil, and add the squash followed by the coconut milk.

4) Add some additional flavoring when you add the turmeric, pepper, and salt.
5) Blend using an immersion blender or a standing blender if you prepare the mixture in batches. The texture should be creamy smooth.

Garnish the way you like it.

Freeze what you don't eat in an air-tight container for up to 6 months.

Note: How to Prepare the Squash: Cook the squash in the slow cooker for 6 hours using the low setting or for 3 hours using the high setting. Let it cool before you cut it in half and discard the peel.

You can also roast it in the oven (cut in halves) for 45 minutes to one hour at 425°F. Discard the seeds.

Yields: 2 to 4 servings

Suitable for vegetarians & vegans

Snacks & Sauces

Baked Turmeric Plantain Chips

These treats are one source full of potassium, Vitamins A, and C, as well as a rich source of dietary fiber. These promote the growth of good bacteria and are resistant to starch as well.

Ingredients
2 plantains (about ½ pound) green plantains
½ tsp. ground turmeric
¼ tsp. ground coriander
½ tsp. salt (or himalayan salt)
¼ tsp. each ground cumin
1 Tbsp. melted sustainable red palm oil

Directions
1) Heat the oven in advance to 350°F.
2) Peel the plantains, but realize the peeling is thick and woody. Use a sharp knife and cut off the top. Slice along the sides to remove the peel. Slice it on an angle.
3) Pour the oil in a dish and coat the plantains.
4) Combine the spices in another bowl and roll the oily plantain through the mixture.
5) Place in a baking dish and bake for 15 minutes; turn them over and continue baking for approximately 10 additional minutes.

6) Transfer the chips from the oven to a cooling rack.
7) Continue until the cycle is completed.
8) Enjoy when the chips have cooled.

Store the finished product in the freezer for no longer than a month. The chips will be fine on the counter for 2 days.

Yields: 1 to 2 servings
Preparation Time: 5 minutes
Cooking Time: 35 to 40 minutes (depending on the thickness)

Suitable for vegetarians & vegans

Rocket Fuel Dry Fruits

Once you try out this recipe, you will understand why it is called rocket fuel, you will really get going.

Ingredients

3 large heaping Tbsp. turmeric
1 cup (300 ml) coconut oil
Pepper and salt
Dry fruits used:
- Cashews
- Walnuts
- Cranberries
- Almonds
- Pomegranate seeds

Directions

1) Use a pan to heat the coconut oil.
2) Add the turmeric.
3) Toss in the fruits and stir.
4) Final stage: Add the pepper and salt to your liking.

Yields: 1 to 2 servings

Suitable for vegetarians & vegans

Tasty Yogurt and Turmeric

Preparing yogurt for a snack or breakfast is a superb way to consume some of your intake of turmeric. Directions do not get much easier than these.

Directions
1) Make a cup of yogurt.
2) Add a teaspoon of turmeric on the top and drizzle with some honey.
3) Combine for a real treat!

Yields: 1 serving

Suitable for vegetarians & vegans

Turmeric Chocolate and Coconut Truffles

Who said you can't enjoy some tasty chocolatey turmeric treats?

Ingredients
½ cup coconut oil
5 Tbsp. maple syrup or raw honey
½ cup raw cocoa powder
1 pinch of salt
1 to 2 tsp. turmeric powder
¼ cup raw shredded coconut

Directions
1) Use a double boiler or create one by using a heat-proof container such as a glass measuring cup over the top a pan of water. Add the coconut oil and allow it to melt slowly.
2) Whisk in the liquid sweetener and cocoa powder until you create a thick - smooth ganache/filling.
3) You can place it in the freezer for a quicker set or place it in a bowl in the refrigerator for about 1 hour.
4) *Make the Coating*: Use a food processor to mix the turmeric and coconut together until it is a bright yellow. Adjust the turmeric to your liking. Add to a bowl.
5) Once the filling is set, roll the mixture — 1 teaspoon at

a time—into a ball and dip it into the coconut mix.
6) Place the batch into the fridge for at least 30 minutes before time to eat them. Enjoy your turmeric filled treat!

These will be okay in the refrigerator for up to five days.

Yields: 2 to 4 servings

Suitable for vegetarians & vegans

Homemade Turmeric Mustard

If you like mustard, you can make this from scratch and keep everyone healthier.

Mix the following ingredients:
- 2 tbsp. white vinegar
- ½ cup ground mustard
- 1 tsp. each salt and turmeric
- 1 tbsp. of water

Store the mustard in a tight-fitting glass jar in the refrigerator.

Turmeric Hummus

This delight is one of the most powerful as well as easy to make cancer-fighting recipes you will find on the 'homemade' scene.

Ingredients
½ cup olive oil
2 (15 ounce) cans drained chickpeas (save ½ cup of the liquid)
1 tsp. sesame oil
4 tsp. minced clove of garlic
1/3 cup lemon juice
2 tsp. turmeric
2 tsp. paprika
¼ tsp. pepper
¾ tsp. salt

Directions
1) Mix the reserved chickpea liquid with the rest of the ingredients using a food processor for about 1 minute.
2) You can add more liquid if desired until you reach the consistency you want.

You can also imagine dipping it with some pita bread or with some veggies. Yummy!

Chapter 5: Turmeric Rich Warm Beverages

Consuming turmeric rich beverages are a great way to quickly absorb the benefits that this amazing spice has to offer. Many of the warm drinks recipes are used specifically to remedy general feelings of being unwell. You must give these a try because they really work wonders.

Warm Drinks

Turmeric Tea Golden Milk Recipe

Have a cup of this recipe to soothe away the aches and pains of the day.

Ingredients
1 tsp. turmeric
2 cups pecan, coconut, or almond milk
½ tsp. cinnamon
Pinch of black pepper (to increase absorption)
¼ tsp. ginger powder or small piece fresh-peeled fresh ginger

Optional
1 pinch of cayenne pepper
1 tsp. raw honey or maple syrup

Directions
1) Prepare all of the components until smooth in a blender (high-speed).
2) Empty the mixture into a pan and heat for about 3 to 5 minutes. (Use medium heat but do not boil the tea.)

Drink and try to enjoy; it is good for you.

Yields: 2 Servings

Turmeric Tea Mix

If you want to have plenty of tea on hand, you can make it in advance. Combine each of these ingredients ahead of time so you can receive the benefits quickly.

Ingredients
¼ cup cinnamon powder
2 tsp. ground black pepper
½ cup turmeric powder
1 to 2 Tbsp. ground ginger

Optional:
½ tsp. of cayenne pepper

Directions
1) When you are ready for a cup, add 2 cups of milk and 2 teaspoons of the mixture.

Yields: 2 Servings

Apple and Green Turmeric Tea
(Cold and Flu Tonic)

Spice up your green tea with a touch of turmeric and apples.

Ingredients
1 large fuji apple (wedges)
4 ½ cup of spring or purified water
1 (2-inch) knob of turmeric or 1 tsp. turmeric powder
2 ceylon cinnamon sticks
1 (2-inch) knob of ginger
1/8 tsp. black pepper
2 tsp. virgin coconut oil
½ tsp. pure vanilla extract
2 Tbsp. fresh lemon juice
1/8 tsp. cayenne pepper
2 organic green tea bags
2 Tbsp. raw honey

Directions
1) Cut the knob of turmeric and ginger into chunks.
2) Use a saucepan over a medium-high setting to bring the water to a boil while adding the vanilla, cayenne, black pepper, apple wedges, ginger, turmeric, coconut oil, and cinnamon sticks.
3) Lower the heat and let it cook (on low) for approximately 30 minutes. Toss the tea bags in and

stir to cook slowly for 3 to 5 more minutes.
4) Discard the bags, and add your lemon juice and honey.
5) Strain the tea into your heat-proof container and pour four servings.

Yields: 4 servings

Turmeric Coffee

If you like your coffee strong, this is perfect to give you a jump start to your day.

Ingredients
½ tsp. ground cinnamon
8 ounces' strong coffee
1 Tbsp. grass-fed unsalted butter
3/8 tsp. ground turmeric
½ tsp. MCT oil
Optional: Raw honey

Directions
1) Brew the coffee with the turmeric and cinnamon.
2) Empty the coffee along with the honey, oil, and butter into a blender.
3) Process until creamy smooth and enjoy.

Yield: 1 serving

Honey and Turmeric Latte

With just a touch of honey, you can bring your latte to life with this fabulous beverage.

Ingredients for the Tea Base
2 chai black tea bags
3 cups boiling water
1 tsp. ground turmeric
1/8 tsp. sea salt
3 Tbsp. raw honey

Ingredients for the Milk
½ cup cashews plus two cups of water blended at high-speed / OR 2 cups homemade cashew milk

Optional:
Ice cubes

Directions
Place the tea bags and boiling water in a glass container to steep for at least 15 to 20 minutes.
1) Discard the tea bags. Whisk in the sea salt, honey, and turmeric while the tea is still warm.
2) Pour the tea base into the glass and top it off with ¼ - ½ cup of the cashew milk.

Yields: 4 servings

Turmeric Hot Chocolate

A bit of hot chocolate can top off a hectic day, and adding turmeric to the mix makes it even better!

Ingredients
8 ounces hot (not boiling) coconut milk or water
2 Tbsp. cocoa powder
1/2 teaspoon turmeric powder

Optional:
- 1 Tbsp. gelatin powder
- 1 tsp. maca powder
- ½ tsp. cinnamon powder
- 1 tsp. honey/maple syrup/stevia drops
- ½ tsp. vanilla extract
- 1 Tbsp. coconut oil/butter

Directions
Mix all of the ingredients in a blender; turn it on and serve warm.

Yields: 1 serving

Spiced Matcha Latte

Spice up your latte with this great mixture of ingredients!

Ingredients
1 tsp. matcha powder
1/8 tsp. ginger
3 ounces boiled water
1/8 tsp. turmeric
¼ tsp. cinnamon
8 ounces warmed non-dairy milk of your choice (or standard dairy milk)
1 drop of stevia (or your choice of natural sweetener)

Directions
1) Prepare the water to a boil in a pan or the microwave. Add part of it to a small glass mixing cup.
2) Blend in the remainder of the ingredients — minus the milk for now — and combine.
3) Add the milk in a large mug and mix with the rest of ingredients; whisk again.
4) Add the sweetener of choice and relax.

Note: This can also be prepared with a NutriBullet blender or similar.

Yields: 1 Serving

Chapter 6: Shakes and Smoothies

Raspberry Collagen Turmeric Shake

Raspberries are natural good for you, so these shakes will be exceptionally tasty with the addition of a banana and the blend of turmeric.

Ingredients
1 large banana
1 cup frozen raspberries
½ tsp. turmeric powder
Pinch of salt
1 Tbsp. lemon juice
½ cup water
2 Tbsp. collagen hydrolysate
1 cup coconut milk

Directions
1) Peel and roughly chop the banana.
2) Put all of the components into a high-speed blender until smooth.
3) Add a splash or so of water if it is too thick.

Yields: 4 small or 2 large glasses

Tropical Turmeric Smoothie

This combination of tasty ingredients will assist the turmeric benefits and get your day off to a great start.

Ingredients
1 large carrot
2 oranges
1/2 cup mango chunks (frozen)
1 Tbsp. raw hemp seeds
2/3 cup coconut water
1 ½ tsp. turmeric
¾ tsp. ginger
Pinch cayenne pepper

Directions
1) Peel and remove the pith of the orange. Scrub and coarsely chop the carrot.
2) Use the ice crush setting/smoothie setting to puree the carrots, orange, cayenne, turmeric, hemp seeds, coconut water, mango, ½ cup of ice, and salt in a blender.
3) Mix until smooth and enjoy!

Yields: 1 large glass

Mango Turmeric Smoothie

The combination of coconut and mango bring the effects of the turmeric front and center to fix whatever is ailing you.

Ingredients
1 cup mango
1 ½ cups water
½ cup coconut flakes (unsweetened and toasted)
1 Tbsp. coconut oil
1 scoop raw plant-based protein powder
1 Tbsp. golden flax seeds
½ tsp. cinnamon
2 tsp. turmeric
2 cm (.8 of an inch) of cubed ginger

Directions
1) Pour all of the ingredients into a blender and combine until creamy smooth.

Yields: 1 serving

Turmeric Ginger Limeade

Add a bit of a kick to your limeade with the addition of turmeric.

Ingredients

1 tsp. dried or 1 (two-inch) - chunk turmeric
3 Tbsp. raw honey
1 (two-inch) piece ginger/1 tsp. dried
½ cup fresh squeezed lime juice
2 cups filtered water

Directions
1) Squeeze 2 to 3 limes for the juice.
2) Peel and cut the turmeric and ginger into 5 or 6 chunks. Place them in four cups of water — bringing it to a boil.
3) Lower the burner's heat, and continue cooking slowly for about five minutes.
4) Turn the heat off. Add the honey; stirring to mix — let it cool.
5) Remove the turmeric and ginger.
6) Use a large canning jar or container to store the drink.
7) Add the last 2 cups of water along with the lime juice.
8) Enjoy right away with a few ice cubes or place it in the fridge for later.

Yields: 2 glasses

Chapter 7: Quick-Fix Turmeric Beauty Mixtures

The benefits of turmeric are boundless, but these are just a few of the basic ones that will provide you with healthier hair and skin. Overall, the elasticity of your skin can be improved with the use of the turmeric because it contains so many antioxidants that it will help stimulate new cell growth.

Healthy Hair and Skin

Anti-Bacterial: Turmeric paste is a superb agent to place on small burns and cuts to help keep bacterial infections away. Apply a small amount of the powder to some aloe vera gel and combine.

Control the Facial Hair: Sometimes, as women age, facial hair growth can become an issue. Turmeric comes to the rescue to slow down or possibly stop the growth of hair. It may not work on men's facial hair because it is usually too thick. All you need is 1 tablespoon of gram flour and ¼ tablespoon of turmeric powder.
Mix the ingredients together and massage it onto your face with wet fingers using a circular motion, which will help pull off the unwanted hair. If you have oily skin; it

is okay to exfoliate up to 3 times weekly. However, only do this once or twice each week if you have dry to normal skin.

Use as a Mask or Wash

Age catches up with everyone at some point in time, but there is no reason to believe you have to give into the decline of your beauty. Fight it with turmeric.

All-Purpose Mask: Add one teaspoon each of honey, turmeric powder and plain yogurt or milk. You can leave it on for no longer than 20 to 30 minutes. Rinse with lukewarm water.

For Wrinkles: Use a combination of rice powder, turmeric, tomato juice, and raw milk to make a paste. Apply and leave it on your face for 30 minutes and wash the pack away with lukewarm water.

For the Aging Lines: Combine some yogurt or milk with some turmeric powder. Apply it using a circular motion, allowing it to dry, and wash off with warm water.

For Acne:

- *Method 1:* Use a face mask made of lime juice, sandalwood powder, and turmeric.
- *Method 2:* You can also try 1 teaspoon each of chickpea powder, turmeric powder, a touch of water, and 1 tablespoon of lemon juice.

Leave the mixture on for ten minutes and wash away with lukewarm water.

For Acne Scars: Prepare a mixture of water and turmeric to a paste and place it on your face for about 15 minutes.

You can also use ½ teaspoon of turmeric, 2 tablespoons of gram flour (also called besan which is a ground chickpea flour), and 3 tablespoons of yogurt. Apply the pack to your face until it dries entirely. Wash it away with some cold water.

Stubborn Zits: Mix some honey with ½ teaspoon of turmeric and a few drops of lemon juice. Apply the mixture to your infected areas and let it stay on for about 20 minutes or so. Wash the mask off with warm water; then a bit of cold water to reduce the size of the pores.

As a Moisturizer: This combination works well for the neck and face area.

- *Method 1*: Use 2 pinches of turmeric with some rosewater and honey. You will feel the difference! Rinse it off when dried.
- *Method 2*: You can also use 2 drops of olive oil, a pinch of turmeric, 1 egg white, rosewater, and fresh lemon juice to the elbows, knees, as well as the neck, and face. Let it dry and rinse away.
- *Method 3*: Combine 1 tablespoon of fresh cream, ½ teaspoon turmeric powder, and 1 tablespoon rosewater. Leave it on for about 30 minutes and rinse away.

An Overnight Cream: Use a combination of yogurt or milk with some turmeric powder (the amount depends on your cream thickness preference). Leave it on all night while you sleep. You can do this about 2 to 3 times each week to recover some younger looking skin.

For Oily Skin: If you suffer from oily skin then this will be great for you to try. Use 1 tablespoon gram flour, ½ teaspoon turmeric powder with a touch of water and touch of freshly squeezed orange juice. Use the paste for about 10 minutes on your face and wash it off using some warm water.

For a Refreshed Face: Make a paste of 1 tablespoon of turmeric, sandalwood powder, neem, and tulsi leaves. Leave the paste on for 30 minutes and rinse.

Dark Circles under the Eyes: Add 2 tablespoons of buttermilk along with a pinch of turmeric in a bowl. Add the paste under your eyes for about 20 minutes. Use fresh water to rinse and close the pores.

Turmeric as a Foundation: Your skin can receive a natural color. The powder can adjust your foundation to match peach, olive, golden, or yellow undertones.

Lighten Pigmentation: Combine a tablespoon of honey, a tablespoon of turmeric, and some mashed papaya. Apply it to your face and let it set for about 20 minutes and wash it away.

Cracked Heels and Skin: Make a paste using some coconut/castor oil and some turmeric powder. Use on the heels or other areas where dry skin is a problem.

Words of Caution

Before you decide to use turmeric creams, you should be diligent and know it can temporarily dye your skin. It is advisable to test an inconspicuous area of your body before you use it on your face.

If you do want to remove the stain, you can use a facial toner or make one using some water and sugar. You can make your personal toner using 1 egg white, 1/3 teaspoon of turmeric powder, and 1 tablespoon of oats. You can also use a cotton ball to help absorb the yellowish coloring.

Chapter 8: Beautiful Homemade Skin Treatments

You know how many ways the packs can help your skin. Now it is time to uncover more precise methods of taking care of *you* using more intense and specific guidelines and recipes.

Neck Area Concoction #1:
Gram Flour, Cream and Turmeric Pack

Ingredients
2 tsp. gram flour
1 tsp. cream
1 tsp. sandalwood
1 pinch of turmeric

Optional: olive oil (or almond oil)

Directions
1) Combine all of the ingredients; unless you have very dry skin, you can add a few drops of olive or almond oil.
2) Blend them to form a smooth paste while making sure there are no lumps formed.
3) Apply to your neck and face for 15 minutes and rinse with warm water.

You can use this if you choose up to 2 or 3 times each week.

Face Cleanse Concoction #2: Turmeric, Almond and Milk Pack

Ingredients
1 tsp. turmeric powder
1 tsp. almond powder
1 tsp. milk

Directions
Mix all of the ingredients to make a paste. If it is too thick, you can adjust with a bit more milk.
1) Apply evenly to clean skin and leave on for approximately 15 to 20 minutes.
2) Use a warm cloth to remove the paste. Lastly, have a splash of cold water.
3) Use this about once each week.

Blackheads Concoction #3: Turmeric and Egg White

Ingredients
½ tsp. rose water
1 tsp. almond oil (or olive oil)
½ tsp. lemon juice
1 egg
½ tsp. turmeric

Directions
1) Begin by mixing a few drops of oil with the egg white.
2) Add the remainder of ingredients.
3) Blend well and keep it on until totally dried and rinse away with some warm water.

You can use this three or four times weekly.

Acne Concoction #4:
The Acne Prone Skin Pack

Ingredients
1 tsp. fuller's earth (i.e. multani mitti)
2 tsp. yogurt
½ tsp. turmeric
½ tsp. rosewater

Optional: 1 tsp. Sandalwood powder

Directions
1) Combine the multani mitti, the pinch of turmeric and yogurt.
2) You can add the sandalwood if you desire an astringent.
3) Blend the chosen ingredients into a paste and spread it over your face.
4) Let it work for about 15 minutes and rinse with some cool water.
5) Do this weekly to help with the acne outbreaks.

Deep Cleaner Concoction#5:
Lemon Juice, Turmeric and Gram Flour

Ingredients
½ tsp. lemon juice
½ tsp. turmeric
2 tsp. gram flour

Directions
1) Mix all of the ingredients into a paste. Add the mixture to your face and let it rest for about 10 to 15 minutes.
2) Rinse, pat your face dry, and follow up the procedure with some moisturizer.
3) You can use the mixture several times each week for a month.

Note: if you have pale skin; be careful you skin could become yellow.

Oily & Dry Skin Concoction #6:
Turmeric, Honey and Cornstarch Pack

This one works for oily and dry skin:

Dry Skin: ½ Tablespoon of almond, olive, or coconut oil

Oily Skin: ½ teaspoon lemon juice and ¼ cup yogurt

Also:

Ingredients
2 Tbsp. cornstarch
A few drops of honey
¼ tsp. turmeric powder

Directions
1) Combine the cornstarch and turmeric into a paste and add the honey to the mix.
2) For the dry skin; you will add the oil to make the paste
3) For the oily skin; the process will use the yogurt and lemon juice to make a creamy mixture.
4) Proceed with the mask on your neck and face for fifteen to twenty minutes.
5) Remove the mask with a warm wet cloth.
6) You can use this once weekly.

If you wonder why it works so well; it is because of the antioxidants in the honey to make your skin glow. The corn starch is the binding that holds the pack together.

Ultimate Face Lift Concoction #7:
The Ultimate Turmeric Face Pack

This face remedy is the leader of the pack! You know how it is sometimes when you have that dull—kind of lifeless look. This pack may be the answer to heal the cells and get you back on track.

Ingredients
¼ tsp. turmeric powder
2 strands good quality saffron
2 Tbsp. carrot juice
2 tsp. honey
½ tsp. lemon juice
½ tsp. almond oil
1 tsp. aloe vera gel
1 tsp. yogurt
1 tsp. glycerin
1 tsp. rosewater
1 tsp. radish juice
1 tsp. powdered gram flour or oats

Directions
1) Blend all of the above components. You can add the gram flour or powdered oats if you do not think your mask will maintain a thick enough consistency.
2) Cream the face pack on, and let it set for twenty

minutes.
3) Take the mask off with a warm rag and a splash or two of cold water.
4) This mixture is good for once a week for about one month.

Cooling Off Concoction #8:
Chill Out with Fuller's Earth

This simple mask of fresh water, ¼ teaspoon of turmeric powder, and 1 tablespoon of Multani Mitti (Fuller's Earth) are the only ingredients needed. Leave it on for 10 to 15 minutes and wash it away. This concoction is a perfect remedy if you live in a hot climate to achieve a relaxed and 'cool' feeling.

Itchy Skin Concoction #9:
Turmeric and Oatmeal Aids Irritation

Mix ½ teaspoon powder, with some water, along with one tablespoon of lentil powder and oatmeal.

This remedy is super for some quick relief of poison ivy or sunburn. Just about any skin irritation is covered as well as the oatmeal is a natural moisturizer.

Dandruff Concoction #10: Dandruff Treatment

Use a combination of olive oil and turmeric on your scalp before taking your shower. Leave the mixture activated and wash your hair with a natural shampoo. The hair follicles will receive nutrition while the increased circulation will clear away any dandruff issues.

Toothpaste Concoction #11: Amazing Turmeric Toothpaste

A study performed by *the Indian Society of Periodontology* found turmeric as a mouthwash beneficial. The spice was extremely useful while preventing gingivitis, plaque build-ups, and noticeable improvements on the anti-inflammatory and anti-microbial properties.

The virgin coconut oil is a natural tooth whitener which makes it the perfect partner for turmeric. These ingredients are the secret:

Ingredients
1 to 2 drops peppermint oil
1 tsp. turmeric powder

1 Tbsp. virgin coconut oil

You can make more if you wish, and it will last for months if you store it in a jar with a tight-fitting lid.

Directions
1) Combine all of the ingredients to form a thick paste.
2) Use as you normally do with any toothpaste.
3) Leave the mixture on your teeth for about three to five minutes.
4) Spit, rinse, and walk away knowing you have a *clean* mouth.

Note: It will not whiten cosmetic teeth or dentures. It's truly amazing how turmeric can whiten your teeth, yet stain other surfaces it touches. The improvements should be noticeable within several days of use.

Conclusion

Thank for viewing each chapter of your personal copy of the *Turmeric Superfoods*. Let's hope it was informative and provided you with a ton of valuable information about the wonderful spice. As you now see, there are so many ways you can use turmeric to remain healthy.

The next step involves deciding which ways you want to begin, whether it is a tasty new drink or a food dish; you can believe it will perform and exceed your expectations. The information you have absorbed can very well change the rest of your life.

Turmeric is probably one of the most versatile spices you can acquire, which has dated back for centuries in Chinese medicine and ancient Indian medicine amongst others. Even though there has not been a huge amount of human research in the field, the evidence is mounting with most of the research provided from curcumin (its active component). And not to forget the thousands, if not millions, of stories of people who have benefited from using it.

In essence, how can you go wrong with all of its proven benefits provided by patients who have received remarkable relief by adding turmeric into their lives? Start adding turmeric into your life today and see how well it can work for you.

Finally, if you found this book useful in any way, leaving a review on Amazon will help this book reach a lot more people and, in turn, help change more lives for the better!

Don't forget to grab your FREE eBook gift before you leave

Click on the link below to get your eBook now...

http://bit.ly/myvouchgift

101 Inspirational Cooking Quotes

Inside this free eBook, you will find amazing cooking tips from famous awe-inspiring people who love to cook just like me and you!

Ps. Feel free to share this free gift with your friends & family!

'Index' on next page...

Index

Introduction

Chapter 1: What is Turmeric?

- Where does Turmeric originate from?
- Chemical Composition of Turmeric
- Ways to Use Turmeric
- Curcumin Elements
- Turmeric Root vs. Powder
- Possible Side Effects

Chapter 2: How Turmeric Helps

- Ailments that Benefit from Turmeric
- Health Benefits in Comparison
- The Research Says It All

Chapter 3: Turmeric 'Golden Paste' Medicinal Remedies

- How to Prepare the 'Golden Paste'
- Daily Supplement Booster
- Additional Ways to Use the 'Golden Paste'
- Benefits for Horses & Pets

Chapter 4: Turmeric Cookbook Recipes

- Breakfast Recipes
    - Turmeric and Onion Omelet
    - Persian Herb Frittata
- Chicken Recipes
    - Coconut Turmeric Chicken
    - Ginger Turmeric Chicken
    - Curried Chicken Pasta Salad
- Beef Recipes
    - Spiced Zucchini Beef
    - Original Beef Curry
- Side Dishes, Soups and Salads
    - Freestyle Rice Using Turmeric Paste
    - Turmeric Barley-Arugula Salad
    - Turmeric Rice
    - Skillet Gnocchi with White Beans and Turmeric
    - Roasted Turmeric Cauliflower
    - Spicy Turmeric Lentils for Salads and Wraps
    - Turmeric Butternut Squash Soup
- Snacks and Sauces
    - Baked Turmeric Plantain Chips
    - Rocket Fuel Dry Fruits
    - Tasty Yogurt and Turmeric
    - Turmeric Chocolate and Raw Coconut Truffle

- Homemade Turmeric Mustard
- Turmeric Hummus

Chapter 5: Turmeric Rich Warm Beverages

- Turmeric Tea Golden Milk Recipe
- Turmeric Tea Mix
- Apple and Green Turmeric Tea (Cold and Flu Tonic)
- Turmeric Coffee
- Honey and Turmeric Latte
- Turmeric Hot Chocolate
- Spiced Matcha Latte

Chapter 6: Shakes and Smoothies

- Raspberry Collagen Turmeric Shake
- Tropical Turmeric Smoothie
- Mango Turmeric Smoothie
- Turmeric Ginger Limeade

Chapter 7: Turmeric Quick-Fix Beauty Remedies

- Your Healthy Hair and Skin
- Use as a Mask or Wash
- Words of Caution

Chapter 8: Beautiful Homemade Skin Treatments

- Neck Area Concoction #1: Gram Flour, Cream and Turmeric Pack
- Face Cleanser Concoction #2: Turmeric, Almond and Milk Pack
- Blackheads Concoction #3: Turmeric and Egg White
- Acne Concoction #4: The Acne Prone Skin Pack
- Deep Cleanser Concoction #5: Lemon Juice, Turmeric and Gram Flour
- Oily and Dry Skin Concoction #6: Turmeric, Honey, and Cornstarch Pack
- Ultimate Face Lift Concoction #7: The Ultimate Turmeric Face Pack
- Cooling Off Concoction #8: Chill Out with Fuller's Earth
- Itchy Skin Concoction #9: Turmeric and Oatmeal Aids Irritation
- Dandruff Concoction #10: Dandruff Treatment
- Toothpaste Concoction #11: Amazing Turmeric Toothpaste

Printed in Great Britain
by Amazon